# BIODYNAMICS OF OSTEOPATHY

## Phase Five

Second Edition

James Jealous D.O.

**For more information about Dr. Jealous please visit:**
**https://BiodynamicsOfOsteopathy.com**

BIODYNAMICS OF OSTEOPATHY Phase Five



Hardback ISBN: 979-8-2955-3928-2

Second Edition 2025

James Jealous D.O. (1943–2021) practiced as an osteopathic physician, teacher and writer for many years. His life's work was to found and develop the specific methodology of Biodynamics of Osteopathy, following the lineage of Dr. A.T. Still and Dr. W.G. Sutherland.

This is one of a series of Biodynamics of Osteopathy books. They grew organically from sets of handouts written by Dr. Jealous and given to students during courses taught by him and his teachers. After many years he collected the handouts together and created individual course manuals, which he added to and rewrote many times. After several more years they evolved further into books.

# TABLE OF CONTENTS

# OSTEOPATHY IS SERVICE

**We use our hands ...**

To treat the Whole patient

To listen to the indwelling movements of Life

To treat all levels of illness

To assist in building the patient's functional reserve

To support homeostasis and trophicity by balancing the activity of the autonomic nervous system

To explore "laws not framed by human hands" (Dr. Still and Dr. Sutherland)

To cooperate and communicate with the Laws of Nature (Dr. Wales)

"To find the Health" (Dr. Still)

To get to the treatment plan

To get to the diagnosis

To help establish a point of Rest or Neutral around which the Whole can come to balance

To find Cause

**We believe ...**

We have an innate capacity to heal
The patient functions as a whole
The autonomic nervous system plays a major role in disease and healing
Structure and function are one form of activity
The Divine is indwelling
Life moves beyond death
There is a Constant Movement toward Normal
We are here to Serve Humanity

**Normal is ...**

"A sense of peace and harmony" (Dr. Sutherland)
Ease of motion, without tension
A capacity for Neutral
A sense of Wholeness to Life
The capacity for adaptation, change without compensation.

**"Skill is proportionate to one's understanding of normal" (Dr. Still)**

*"It is convenient to describe cranial articular mobility in three divisions, but it is necessary to remember that the whole includes the parts, and that the action occurs simultaneously in all parts."*

*W. G Sutherland, D.O. (Teachings in the Science of Osteopathy, p. 67)*

*"I deem it my duty to caution in the usage of any application of a direct contact technique to the basisphenoid or petrous portion apex. This type of technique directly effects a severe strain to the junction area of the great cerebral vein with the straight sinus. Please consider this as a constructive criticism by one who has had considerably more experience than others in the picture. Enough said, I hope."*

*W.G.S.*

*(1949 OCA Journal)*

*"You will train them to observe without interfering."*

*W.G.S.*

*(Teachings in the Science of Osteopathy, p. 151)*

# THE FACE

## *Phase One is about involuntary motion, which is motion present in the Whole and in the lesion.*

In our work we learned to synchronize with the breathing of primary respiration before we approached any treatment. This synchronization is the key to working with stable rates and not irritating the system. This principle of synchronizing with a Healthy aspect of the patient suffuses the whole teaching program. We begin with the Health! This synchronization shifts our awareness to a different level of receptivity, which allows us to see primary respiration rather than the lesion field, and this eventually leads us to an understanding of the intention of primary respiration.

## *Phase Two is about communication with the natural laws of healing that surround activity at two to three cycles per minute.*

In our work in Phase Two, we not only synchronized with the breathing of primary respiration but also added the skill of sensing the fulcrum, the Stillness around and through which the breathing is creating its form and function.

This is a different kind of synchronization from that in Phase One, and it shifted our awareness more deeply.

As this new format occurs, the treatment automatically expresses itself. The end point of treatment, when compared with Phase One, reveals several differences. Stillpoints are deeper and wider, and after the rate returns, it is much slower than in the beginning.

Also, we find that this kind of synchronization works exclusively with the fluid body, and the outcome of treatment is more complete than when working with tissue alone. This is because fluid body dynamics form the tissue, and by working in this way we find tissue is able to be more metabolically stable, a precursor to healing.

At first we do not fully trust it, but later we see the truth and wisdom of this method and how it fits with the explanations of Sutherland and Still. (Reread the first chapter of *Philosophy of Osteopathy* by A. T. Still.)

## *Phase Three is centered around the activities of the Long-Tide, which is where Phase Two ended.*

In Phase Three we explored a therapeutic force already present in the lesion field.

We looked at the "sacs" of the cranium. We learned that the dural system is not made up of three sickles, but rather a series of folds in a sac, arising during growth and development. We saw the amazing relationship between the upper and lower dural sacs, one around the brain proper and one around the cerebellum. This awakened us to the independence of two separate tents.

We found also that the Long-Tide is an expression of the "Sea Around Us." We noted that Zone D, the horizon, and the Wire (along which the Long-Tide moves during its intended therapeutic course) are all linked as natural laws pertaining to this level of Primary Respiration (100 seconds per cycle). For us to synchronize with this level, we needed to be aware of an Ocean the size of the circumference of the horizon, to exhale our attention, and to wait. This reveals another pathway to another level of the Tide. Importantly, we saw that the Long-Tide cannot be approached without the above knowledge, which took many years to explore and begin to understand.

### *Phase Four focuses on the midline.*

The midline synchronizes us. It centers us in such a way that we become naturally aware of Zone D and the dynamic stillness in the "Sea Around Us." This is not Zone A, Zone B, or the Long-Tide. The midline is not a line but a place where the spatial relationships are expressed as a whole ... it is not like the segmental embryology, which centers around the notochord. The Midline is the sanctuary of the Health and its therapeutic forces.

The Stillness in Phase Four is very different from that in the earlier Phases. Here, in this new world, we are centered by the "Stillness at the Center of Creation."

### *Phase Five is a pause, a chance to Breathe.*

As we leave Phase Four behind, we need time to adapt to the Tide Centering Us. This can take years, and often does, because we do not see it happen. It can happen any time of the day or night, and the heart must take it in and see the help very clearly. The Third Level stillness announced in Phase Four is a real truth, and our senses need to appreciate the new terrain.

### *In Phase Five of Biodynamics of Osteopathy we come to the Face.*

I have put this together from watching the Tide take me to a new understanding. I feel like a reporter for the Ocean News.

The treatment of the face was another masterpiece of Will

Sutherland. I am sure you all know the detailed anatomy of the sutures that he introduced into the profession. The face as a biomechanical reality, driven by the base that was driven by the three sickles, was a masterpiece of understanding. The face presented in that way has limits that are effects of the limitations of sutural-oriented direct action technique. Sutherland clearly states many times that he went beyond the model Magoun preferred.

In Phase Four, we studied the dynamic stillness of the midline, and we began to let our senses work without anatomy, segments, or fluid fields. The outcomes in clinical practice are wonderful. The Tide has taken us somewhere. This is how the biodynamics of the face became what it is. We have been brought here by the Stillness that Centers Us.

As we work in this phase, we will use all of the principles that we have learned to date. We will work with automatic shifting (2–3 cpm) and see what that tells us about the face that is different from the older model.

We will work with the therapeutic presence of the Long-Tide and see what we can learn about the face from that landscape.

We will also work with the Dynamic Stillness and see what it teaches us, and, of course, ignition will not be far away from the outcomes.

This could be a review except we must learn a new format and language for the face that better fits our needs as Osteopaths.

# FIRST MEDITATION FOR PHASE FIVE

In Phase Four we observed that the breaths of Primary and thoracic respiration are connected. We sensed each separately while being aware of a Stillness in Zone C. This usually creates a stable attention and opens doors to seeing more about the relationships endemic to respiration.

Now we will explore this further while our hands are on the patient. The search here is for the fulcrum, the birthplace of the common "parent" from which both arise as One.

In Phases Six, Seven, and Eight this will change a lot as we see into the misconceptions we harbor about the primacy of one over the other. We will also see that thoracic respiration is more than the lungs, ribs, and a diaphragm, which is why we started the CV4 exploration. Also, in Phase Four we made a note of the First Breath and the synchronization of Breathing and Ignition as a singularity that increases the vitality of the newborn and the capacity for unfolding.

In ourselves are the answers, not in a book. You are not here to follow me, but rather to see and understand the principles that Osteopathy has given us:

1. Find the health.
2. Where is the fulcrum of the process you are observing?
3. The Tide centers you.
4. Wholeness is the chosen reality of Osteopathy.
5. All this is about you as well as the patient.
6. We are tracking the scent of the Tide; there is no map.
7. Follow what brings your heart and mind ease.
8. Go in the direction of your health.
9. Look for something you've never seen or heard of before.

# OBSERVATION OF THORACIC RESPIRATION

## Practical

Thoracic respiration is not just the somatic movements of the ribs, lungs, and diaphragm.

Breathing is oxygen, metabolism, waste, and renewal in every drop of the whole.

Thoracic respiration is perfect in the health; it moves with no resistance.

All living things are breathing.

Thoracic respiration did not begin with you. It began at the beginning, which is Eternal.

The next breath is the same as the First Breath, breathed into the nostrils of the first Person.

Where is the parent fulcrum upon which the thoracic respiration comes to rest and from which it is formed?

# THE FLUID FIELDS OF THE FACE

This first section is usually a little mind-boggling, probably because embryologists and anatomists have both contributed to our knowledge of the face and have never developed a common language. The names sometimes come from one discipline and sometimes the other. This confuses the practical mind of a clinician who wisely sees the incongruities.

Dr. Sutherland's work on the treatment of the face is yet another model. I hope the reader has had the benefit of studying his detailed discussions of the highly refined and precise sutures of the skull and their movements. There are many ways of looking at the head and upper neck. All of them will interlock in your mind as a single picture once you work with the Biodynamic model and see the images that the Tide brings to you.

Osteopathy is about the Natural Laws of healing. Nothing more. These laws are "not framed by human hands." These words are deeply important; we must follow nature and not the books. We are exploring communication with the Natural world, and we hope to be led by the indwelling therapeutic forces.

***To follow nature is not to lead her.***

This knowledge of following Nature and not manipulating her echoes in Western philosophy all the way back to Socrates, and in the East to the ancient Sanskrit teachings. It has always been the dilemma of the human psyche to break free from its thoughts and listen without bias. This course of action is hard. Just to listen with the hands for something you have never seen before will create friction with self-centering knowledge and popular worldviews. Sutherland went through this process himself (see The Sutherland Perceptual Odyssey, Phase One).

### *We try to "always be beginners" with fresh neutral hearts.*

Our task in the Osteopathic tradition is to dig on, as nature leads. Our core responsibility is to learn to communicate and cooperate with the indwelling capacity of Nature to find a balance point of REST, through which we can find our own inner conversation with the health. This rest is where and when the work of recovery and reorganization occurs. It is a state of complete de-facilitation. This understanding is not new. Both Sutherland and Littlejohn mention John Hilton's book *Rest and Pain*. Hoover as well was on the track of the importance of neutral. Still turned our minds toward it all.

Keep the old knowledge out of the moment and watch. Then let the old and new understandings converge into a new image. This takes a while, so be patient, please. A picture will emerge, then the Tide is teaching you.

The idea of fluid fields is nothing new. It has been a part of embryology and Osteopathy for more than fifty years. The task of putting these two fields together is an original part of the biodynamics contribution to Osteopathy. The information was revealed by the Tide.

The effort to blend the works of Dr. Blechschmidt and Dr. Sutherland was a moment of grace for me. Seeing that two men were aware of the same Mystery, and that they were inspired by Love for Beauty, opened a great doorway.

The similarities in their descriptions still seem almost surreal at times.

The profession was slow to pick up on the message. I believe this is partly because of the mental renovation it requires and the hours of study it demands. We did not put the old wine in new bottles, we put new wine in new bottles.

The work of many people and hard critics has been invaluable in developing this program and its language. Since 1982 the picture has rapidly unfolded and has continued to emerge more quickly as time has passed.

I now realize that I will never see the end of the principle the Tide unveils. The story comes to a point where the future cannot be assumed during treatment. The same treatment never occurs twice.

One must be aware of the Dynamic Stillness that points the way and be free to let oneself be healed as the Tide works.

One thing is certain ... the Breath of Life is always filling the emptiness with Love. Our little cups become one ... then the person who began exploring this work dives into a bigger cup with more Fire.

Please do not try to learn academics. I will repeat things over and over in different styles. Just listen, and watch how much beauty invades your mind. The beauty is alive and it will guide you. The memory will come from love, not study.

My task is to describe and create a language as a means of communication. This will simplify the blending of all disciplines. This is necessary because the languages of different disciplines are not compatible with Osteopathic evaluation and treatment. The outcome will be an easier understanding of all the disciplines and treatment dynamics.

***Form is a mathematically precise event. The accuracy of the Tide is severe. The fulcrum is in the sea. Out of the sea comes formation.***

***The ten-degree logarithmic spiral is the basis of the form.***

The fluid fields create the central nervous system, cranial viscera, and bones. Each segment has neural, visceral, and somatic activities to perform as one symphony in the entire head and upper neck. These fluid fields are not just on the front of the face but all the way through, in a three-dimensional manner.

### *We start with the upper fluid field of the face*

### *The middle fluid field of the face is also known as the maxillary swelling*

### *The lower fluid field of the face is also known as the mandibular arch, the first pharyngeal arch, or the first branchial arch*

The variety of names comes from the archaic theory that humans evolved from fishes. The proof that humans are unique from the moment of conception did not, however, change the terminology, so I have created different language for our purposes. We now have upper, middle, and lower face fluid fields that are capable of growth and development as a whole region of the head, not just the front.

This is an Osteopathic view of the developmental process for the whole head and upper neck, designed to make this biodynamic teaching more easily understood.

This means we abandon the idea of a base, a face, and a vault as the segments of the head.

This view also eliminates the division of the cranium into a neurocranium, a visceral cranium, and an osseous cranium. As you know, these names refer only to bony areas.

The picture we want is one of fluid field segments synchronically working together to express the growth and development of the whole head and upper neck as a unit. This means each fluid field expresses somatic, visceral, and neural functions for its region, much like the segments we find around the notochord. This allows a more Osteopathic bias and develops a language that makes sense to us.

In the past, our profession has looked at the face through local bones, leaving out the wholeness of fluid field dynamics and neuro-visceral activity in the process of growth and healing.

***There is another fluid field held below the lower face fluid field: the hyoid fluid field. It has other names: the second pharyngeal arch, or the second branchial arch***

Our language will be simple. This is not the second arch, it is the fourth, but we will call it the hyoid fluid field, which is below the lower face fluid field. This field extends its fluency through a large area of the whole head and upper neck.

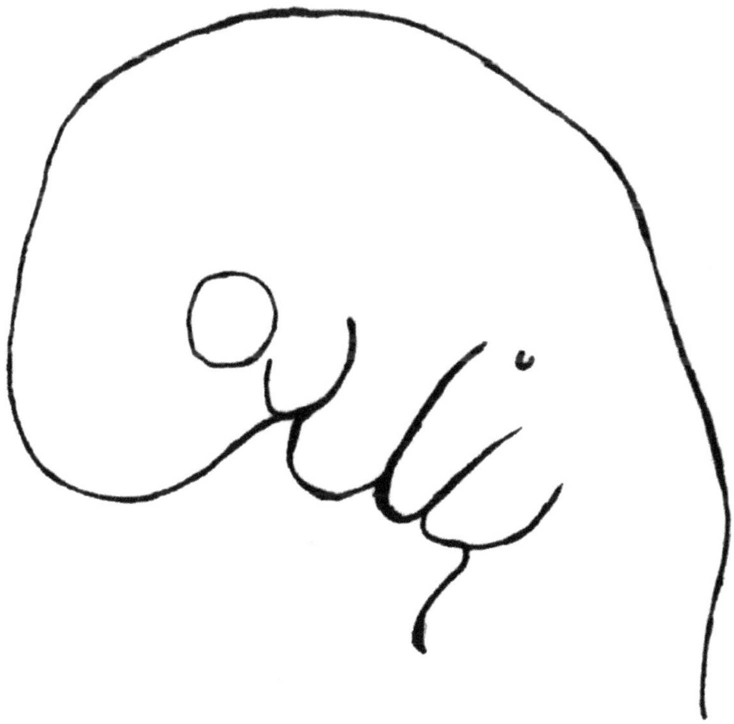

***"There is another field below the hyoid fluid field: the laryngeal fluid field.***

This arch is usually the third arch, but for us it is the fifth. We will call it the laryngeal fluid field.

# PRACTICAL ON THE FACIAL FLUID FIELDS

### *Objectives of this Practical*

One objective is to become aware of the fourth-dimensional motions of Primary Respiration in the Fluid Fields. This may involve breaking habits developed from direct action models, or models with bony or sutural orientation. The habit of having one active and one stabilizing hand while treating must be changed. Our hands are listening and our mind is neutral. Fluid moves in all directions. If our habit is to look from front to back while treating the face, we will shear the fluid by imposing this direction with our attention. The habits, if any, will show up in the practical as we shift our hands many times to see if we have any limitations.

The other objective is to map out the fluid field as you see it. It will be lesioned, so your map will be unique for this patient. We will compare what you find to the ideal healthy model and learn how to interpret what we see.

***When fluid lesions, it locks up and feels like tissue.***

This helps to explain some of the strange tissue-like sensations we will come across in this session. Fluid lesioning has many causes, but to realize the fulcrum where the field is being held will open our eyes to new diagnostics that improve clinical outcomes.

***The Whole will emerge as we progress.***

Here is a diagram of how the fluid fields appear in the head and face.

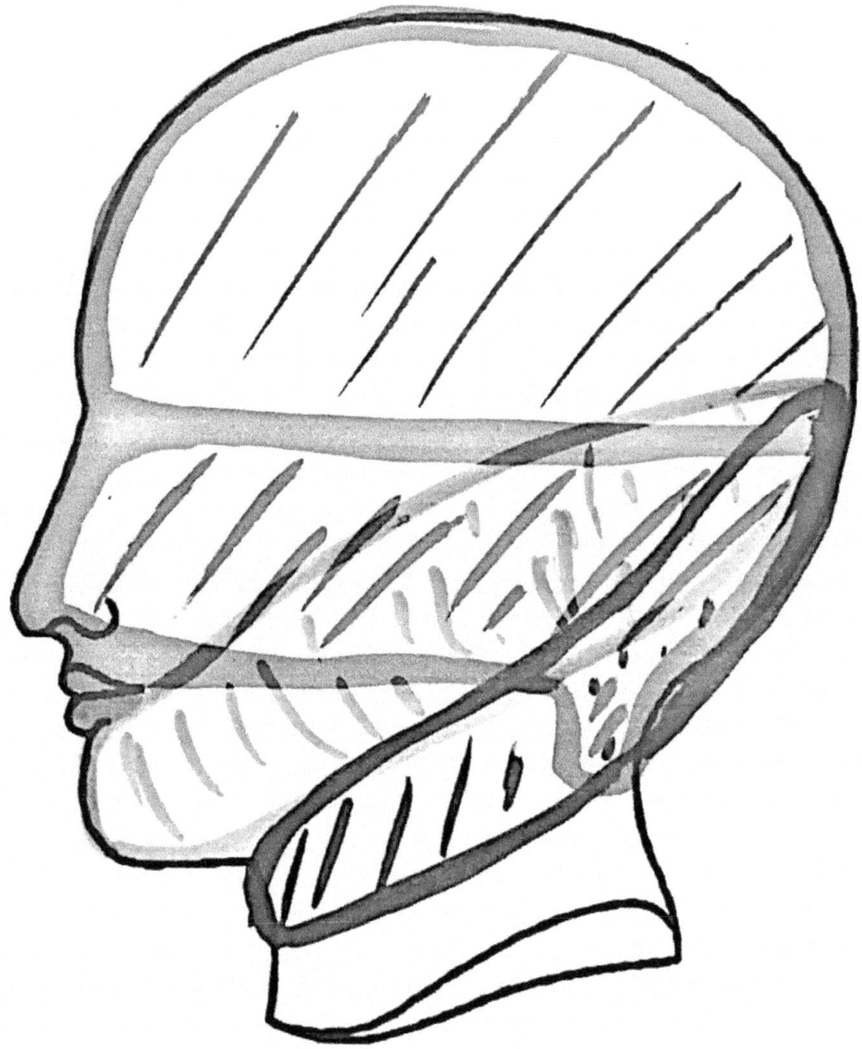

# A COMPARISON OF MECHANICAL AND BIODYNAMIC MODELS OF FACIAL DYNAMICS

***By James Jealous, D.O.***

### *Magoun: No. 1*

The face is moved by the sphenoid under the influence of the falx. The sphenoid passes motive force through the palatines, zygoma, and vomer through interlocking gears and speed reducers. Therefore, the face and the vault are both secondary motions arising from action of the reciprocal tension membrane on the base. The causal forces are mechanical.

### *Biodynamics: No. 1*

The face is moved independently of the base. All tissue, soma, visceral, and neurocranial motions are directly under the influence of the tidal forces of primary respiration.

Motion arises from metabolic activity that is an effect of innate biological transmutation, augmentation, synchronization, and disengagement. Four sutures are seen as doorways that open and close—not gears. Bony motion is not linear mechanics but intraosseous breathing and a changing shape and tone during primary respiration. The underlying principle of motion is the universality of protoplasmic response to primary respiration.

Additionally: In children the gears are not present, so articular gearing from the sphenoid to the face, the manner described for adults, is not probable. The reciprocal tension membrane also (falx cerebri and tentorium cerebelli) is meningeal dural tissue not attached to the periosteum in newborns as in adults. Another explanation for the basis of involuntary motion necessary for growth and development must be considered. The fluid drive in the embryological fields in protoplasm is a more probable rationale.

### *Magoun: No. 2*

The upper face (frontal bone) hangs from the anterior coronal suture of the parietal bones. This is declared as a suspensory force for the upper face.

### *Biodynamics: No. 2*

Suspensory forces are in the fluid field and the potency of the tide. Again, the face in the newborn and young child has no articular surfaces to "hang" from. Also, the bones are not pulled upon by gravity but held in position and poised by fluid and tidal forces.

### *Magoun: No. 3*

The mandible is an unpaired bone.

### *Biodynamics: No. 3*

The mandible is paired throughout life and is similar to the frontal bones with midline sutured motion.

### *Magoun: No. 4*

Facial dysfunction is addressed through the base first. Treatment of the sphenoid first is recommended.

## *Biodynamics: No. 4*

Normalization of fluid drive and its spatial dynamics is a key element in providing normalization of the cranium and its contents. Magoun makes no mention of the motions and principles of treatment other than a mechanical entrapment process that must be addressed with direct action.

## *Magoun: No. 5*

Palatines and maxillaries are the most common lesion sites.

## *Biodynamics: No. 5*

The most common lesion is loss of fluid drive and its ability to express automatic shifting, the constant expression of growth.

## *Magoun: No. 6*

Craniofacial disfigurement and asymmetry is usually secondary to local mechanical lesion.

## *Biodynamics: No. 6*

Regional and Whole fluid body dynamics can lesion the face.

## *Magoun: No. 7*

Treatment of infants uses the following principles:

1. Motion test
2. Direction of ease (usually direction of lesion)
3. Into barrier
4. Hold
5. Articular release between bones at suture is end point

***Patient's cooperation and direction of the tide is mentioned in only one sentence without particulars.***

### *Biodynamics: No. 7*

1. First, reestablish neutral in whole patient.
2. Contact the Stillness in the fluid field.
3. Wait—wait some more.
4. Automatic shifting of therapeutic forces releases bone/membrane/fluid and potency in embryological segment or region.

### *Magoun: No. 8*

Hold one bone, disengage the other (e.g., sphenoid/palatines).

### *Biodynamics: No. 8*

Balanced fluid tension, using motion present inside lesion.

William G. Sutherland in *Contributions of Thought* discusses synchronization before treating, so as to not disturb fluids. Thomas Schooley, in the 1953 *OCA Journal*, recommends balanced fluid tension without using tissue force for molding. Magoun used only repetitive mechanical pressure (e.g., maxillary remolding) for molding intraosseous lesions.

### *Magoun: No. 9*

Relates mandible to temporal bones.

## *Biodynamics: No. 9*

The growth and development of the mandible has influences from the first pharyngeal arch, neurocranial tissues, and occipital tissue forces, etc.

Treatment of the developing mandible involves a very large fluid field that only partially relates to developmental fields in TMJ and embraces the entire midline, head, and upper neck.

## *Magoun: No. 10*

Intraosseous lesions are between embryological parts of bone (petrous, temporal, mastoid temporal, et cetera).

## *Biodynamics: No. 10*

While the lesions described by Magoun do occur as primarily orthopedic events rather than somatic dysfunction, more commonly the whole intraosseous matrix of the bone carries the lesion field, and it crosses articular surfaces. One is not sensing the pieces; one approaches the whole bone and its metabolic relationship between tissue, fluid drive, and biokinetic and biodynamic forces simultaneously so that automatic self-correction can occur in the whole metabolic arena.

## *Magoun: No. 11*

Correct bone.

Wales/Fulford/W.G. Sutherland – balanced membranes, not bones.

### *Biodynamics: No. 11*

Gets the whole released through its own neutral.

### *Magoun: No. 12*

End point of facial treatment is in sutural release from applied forces.

### *Biodynamics: No. 12*

End points are a stillpoint in the whole, not a release of local tissue tensions.

### *Reading:*

*The Ontogenetic Basis of Human Anatomy,* E. Blechschmidt, M.D.
"Fulcrums," T. Schooley, D.O., 1953 *OCA Journal*

# THE FACE

## *More Overview*

In reality, the embryonic head and upper neck are the size of a grape seed.

The whole head and upper neck grow as one space with fluid field segmentations, as we described earlier. The face begins around one month in utero. It finishes (scientifically) around age twenty-eight; however, it continues to renew and heal itself throughout life, using the same indwelling forces as we see in the embryo.

There is a tendency to make treatment about somatic forces; this needs serious reconsideration. Dr. Still, in the first chapter of his *Philosophy of Osteopathy,* is clear about the word anatomy being wholistic and not just somatic.

The language used in basic cranial courses is not developmentally accurate. The word cranium does not include the mandible or the upper neck. The word head does not include the upper neck, which is part of its fluid fields. The words base, face and vault have no meaning in the picture of the developmental movements. They are just bony anatomy, as are the words neuro, viscera, and chondrocranium. The bones do not hang from each other, they are suspended by fluid field forces, which, as we saw in Phase Two, are antigravitational forces. As we move along the road of understanding the facial fluid fields, let's move toward the bigger picture and repair our understandings.

Our goal is to see any limitations we have acquired relative to treatment of the face, cranium, head, and upper neck and to reshape our overview. Several things are important:

The ear is not conditioned by the temporal bone. The ear is an effect of the upper four fluid fields moving toward a predetermined fulcrum, where we see the mature ear. It is not finished positioning itself at birth but settles into adult form only as the adult teeth begin to move. From birth to near age seven, the tympanic membrane faces toward the floor. The treatment of ear problems requires an awareness of all the fluid fields that affect it and the whole of Zone B. Looking only at the temporal bone for ear problems is a serious misunderstanding of growth and development. But adults heal using the same fluid fields. Wholeness is greater than we can imagine. Every change creates a specific positional shift and the effect of a movement in the whole.

The temporal bone is formed from multiple fluid fields, not three internal segments (squamous, petrous, mastoid), which are only a superficial part of the outcome.

The stylohyoid ligament represents the anatomy of two fluid fields, and the inferior surface of the bone is also contributed to by the lower face fluid field and the hyoid fluid field.

To treat the temporal on its theoretical axis as an isolated bone is not accurate and limits the therapeutic potential. All this applies to all cranial bones. The fluid forces that position and heal are much greater than the sutural boundaries.

The eye is an evagination of the third ventricle. The optic chiasm is inside lamina terminalis (the anterior wall of the third ventricle). The muscles of the eye are from the fluid field between the anterior and middle cranial fossae (anterior dural girdle fluid field). The eye is a mini cranium; it has every layer we see in the meninges that we studied in Phase Three. It is not receiving its functions from the orbital cavity, which we might be prone to treat when the eyes are dysfunctional.

In the treatment of head trauma, we first try to reestablish the whole, and then, if necessary, the parts can be addressed through the fluid fields. Rarely is it necessary.

In children, the kaleidoscopic movement in the whole head and upper neck is the foundation of normal neuro-visceral-perceptual-somatic growth in the head and upper neck.

# TREATMENT OF THE FACE
# FIRST LEVEL AUTOMATIC SHIFTING

Automatic shifting is a language used by Dr. Sutherland to describe healthy function. He often referred to suspended automatically shifting fulcrums.

"The Tour of the Minnow" is a story that alludes to this process but does not directly state it. The clearest description of automatic shifting is in an article by Alice Paulsen, D.O., in the 1953 *OCA Journal.* She reports very clearly. Unfortunately, the journal was not known to anyone until Anne Wales gave it to me in 1989. There had never been a teaching about automatic shifting since Will's death, until 1990 when the biodynamic model was introduced.

It took many years of exploration to piece together how one could initiate automatic shifting on demand and what its meaning was in practice. I am still finding it an amazing event. Later, in 1992, it seemed to me that automatic shifting could be the Biokinetics that Blechschmidt refers to in his work.

The outcome for me is this: Biokinetics is less descriptive of the process than what we see osteopathically during treatment. The Biokinetic view does not include the living activity, even though the author sees into the subject deeply. Witnessing the whole repositioning, resynchronizing, and transmuting of the parts is an experience no words can fulfill. The Biokinetics principles are built on the assumption that automatic shifting occurs and is an effect of a Biodynamic force (the Sea Around Us).

What automatic shifting does is prove Osteopathy.

Indwelling therapeutic forces "not framed by human hands" are more than an idea. They can be seen directly, not by inference. This alone is amazing.

The cooperation and communication are from nature to the observer, not the other way around. Nature expresses Osteopathy right before us and we slowly understand the language.

The creation of neutral is a precursor.

The awareness of the whole fluid body as a singularity is necessary; this means segmental or anatomical relationships are not visible during neutral.

Automatic shifting as Paulsen describes it only occurs at two to three cycles per minute. An interesting journey.

As time passed it was obvious that there were several kinds of automatic shifting at different levels of potency (rate related). The picture and power of automatic shifting is unique. For example, the automatic shifting related to the Long-Tide is a much slower, warmer, gel-like continuum than the faster ping-pong-like movements at 2–3 cpm.

The automatic shifting from the Dynamic Stillness moves us first, then unveils a deep connection between the house and the sea. A wave of stillness with intention moves everywhere and suffuses a world with no forms. This is often seen in the care of children.

The power of these Tidal forces provides not just indwelling therapeutics but also diagnostic specifics; one begins to see priorities that are beyond any human capacity. For many years I meticulously compared my diagnostic summary with that of the tide, seeing every time, with rare exceptions, that I overlooked many things. I tried harder. The outcome was no better. We are, when compared to nature's wisdom, frail, uncaring, mental morons. Now I am completely content to follow such a loving, precise, masterful teacher.

It can take some years to appreciate ignorance as a gift.

The Tide begins to teach us the multitude of natural and divine resources awaiting us.

As you work, review the principles in the above commentary to set the stage for the tide to show you its diagnosis.

After the treatment, diagram the automatic shifting and compare it with your diagram.

### *The Treatment*

You already learned the treatment principles in Phase Two:

Establish neutral if necessary.

Then go to the underlying central stillness that connects the sea and Zone B, and wait.

A neutral mind has no sense of why it is waiting.

# AUTOMATIC SHIFTING REVIEW

1. The Neutral Is Vital
2. Automatic Shifting - Fluid Body
    a. Synchronization with Primary Respiration
    b. Tempo of Observer
    c. Precision is Infinite, as is the potential in the moment
    d. Void may not be necessary
3. Therapeutic Forces vs. Effects of Treatment
    a. Stay with therapeutic agencies
    b. Avoid
        i. Compensatory fluid motions
        ii. Barriers
        iii. Therapeutic effects
            1. Last longer than therapeutic input
            2. Tissue motion is always an effect
        iv. Augmentation – we augment through synchronization
    c. Observe the specific and the global

4. The Access
    a. 2–3 cpm
    b. Void
    c. Wait—sense of fluid sea
    d. Minnow appears
    e. May occur without void
5. End Point
    a. Pattern ends at specific site
        i. Notation for next visit

    - ii. Forces recede to midline like a CV4
    - iii. Stillpoint or pause
        1. If pause, may go to Long-Tide then convert to 2–3 cpm
    - iv. Chart pattern of work done by automatic shifting
6. Rebalancing at End of Treatment
    a. We are never a perfect act of conscience

# THORACIC RESPIRATION MEDITATION

The importance of thoracic respiration has transilluminated the history of Osteopathy. The secrets that lay hidden in its chambers are many.

We all learn the gross anatomy of the somatic movements of the thorax that we treat to restore the various limitations that habits and disease may impose on a patient's respiratory effort.

The relationship between the movement of lymph throughout the body and thoracic respiration is another valued truth inherited from our founder, Dr. Still.

Some of us were also trained to look at thoracic respiration as the therapeutic force that carries out the effects of a treatment when the patient returns home (that carries on with the treatment once we have created motion in the tissues).

Dr. Sutherland's teachings mirror an intense understanding of thoracic respiration, neutral, and the capacity of the body to function as a whole. Hoover's work is mentioned by Sutherland often. These were the pioneers of functional treatment, the indirect exaggeration of the lesion motion until a neutral was established that was so whole and quiescent that the diaphragm idled; that is, it moved without resistance.

The therapeutic effects of this freedom in all the fluids and the level of rest it accomplished in the immune system turned away many involuting illnesses.

We know very little about thoracic respiration and its role as a synchronistic force in the well-being of body, soul, and spirit. It is certainly more than just somatic activity. Thoracic respiration is in every cell, every drop, and it is a single movement in the whole. Begin to see how deeply it runs.

Thoracic respiration, when in neutral, moves without resistance. It is as sweet as the breathing of a sleeping newborn!

When the breathing is neutral, in that balance it reconnects with the sea around us and primary respiration, then a pause, then one breath, one breath in the health, one embryonic breath.

Our meditation today is about observing the different levels of breathing in ourselves.

The levels follow the direction of ease, physiological barrier, and anatomical barrier that are traditional to the Osteopathic method.

Our journey will take us to ease, neutral, and the sea; perhaps they will reunite.

# THE SEAMS

As we study the fluid fields of the face, we notice that there are clefts between them. We are going to call these spaces seams, because the embryological words have distinct limitations.

The seams precede the segments; they are there first.

Imagine the protoplasmic embryonic disc that enfolds as a whole, giving rise to an invisible form.

The enfoldments are seams.

If you take a garment off its hanger and drop it on the floor, it enfolds. Seams look like they are effects of abutting fluid fields, but they are not.

The seams are not just in front, as the books suggest, but rather all the way through to the back of the head.

The seams are synchronized by the central midline (see Phase Four) so that all the seams everywhere are trying to be as one movement.

## *The Seams Practical*

This practical involves finding a functional seam of interest and sensing the presence of the Long-Tide.

Because we are in lesion (not perfect), the anatomical seam, the fluid field seam, and the perfect seam of the health are in different locations.

The anatomical seam is found easily.

The functional seam is in another location and is found by scanning.

The health will be studied in Phase Seven.

## *The Treatment*

Find the seam of interest.
Find the Long-Tide in space, not in the space between structures. It feels like an empty, dark room. As the treatment progresses, the seams will merge into a deep darkness (space, again).
Wait.
The ignition will fire somewhere, not necessarily the third ventricle.
Be aware of the whole, so you can see where it happens.
Wait.
Rebalance Zone B with the sea around us.

# THE MIDDLE FACE SEAM

The middle face seam was noticed after the work on the upper, middle, lower, and hyoid fields had been made clear by watching the boundaries established during automatic shifting. The text *Biokinetics and Biodynamics of Human Differentiation* showed that the zygomatic and maxillary arches were separate fluid fields. From this and several insights from the Tide, it became clear that there was a seam between them.

After this information was used in diagnosis and treatment, it became clear that this was an important place. Further study revealed that this seam is related to the dental arch, tooth eruption, and the maxillary sinuses.

This seam in the middle fluid field is vital to the fullness of the vertical height of the middle face. In Down syndrome it needs attention. It is often compressed. It can involute. So spend time with it in practice.

# THE MIDDLE FACE FLUID FIELD

This topic is exceptional. Enjoy it.

The middle face fluid field is below the upper and above the lower facial fluid field.

But it extends all the way to the area of the third cervical vertebra (C3).

It is synchronized with the pelvis in a remarkable manner.

The tissues, viscera, and neural elements are far-reaching.

In a newborn, it is short and the baseline almost flat.

In the adult, it is at full height and the base has a 125-degree angle (sphenobasilar symphysis).

In the adult, it curves from premaxilla to C3 like a banana, so we call it "the banana."

From birth to age twenty-eight, this movement of creating a curvature is life-sensitive. That means that this fluid field must be neutral enough to allow this curvature to occur in the cranial base and brainstem. If it does not flex, the foramen magnum will not change shape, resulting in pressure on the spinal cord and brainstem, causing neurological issues.

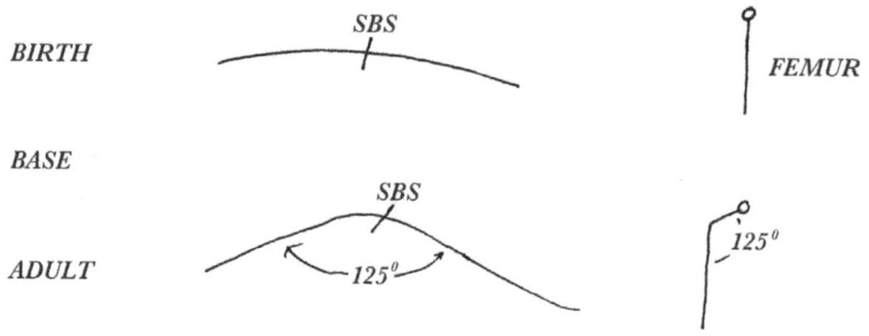

The developing clivus depends on this fluid field to express its angulation. The cerebellum, likewise, needs its shape to change, as does the brainstem all the way to the C3 area. Motor skills develop with this curvature, so we can see here that the internal matrix of the central nervous system is also curving, widening and increasing in vertical height. The venous sinuses are changing their shapes, as are the meninges, and the bones are changing in size. Note that the squamous occiput is in the upper field and the supraocciput is in the middle field. The upper tent is in the upper field and the lower tent is in the middle field. Frank Willard told me that the cerebellum grows eight times faster than the cerebrum in a newborn. This means that the occipital bone is under the influence of two fields, and so we should not look at the squamous occiput as one but rather two areas of the occiput with markedly different inputs during childhood.

The middle face fluid field has a synchronized relationship with the pelvis. Remember, there is no distance in the mind of the fluid body.

As the sinuses in the head grow (along with the rest), the sigmoid sinus that was straight at birth becomes sigmoidal. It curves in one plane as the clivus curves in another plane, both moving toward 125-degree angulation. Meanwhile, the master mechanic is following the same blueprint and curving the femurs.

The femurs are straight at birth. Over the first year, they begin to curve, creating an angle between the femoral neck and the shaft until 125 degrees is reached. As this happens, the transverse diameter widens in the pelvic fluid fields and the bladder descends. These changes are synchronistic with the middle face changes. As one pediatrician said on learning this, "I always wondered why bladder control and gross motor development (cerebellum) were so connected in their onset."

The more we understand the wholeness of this process, the easier it will be to become aware of the parts and the whole together.

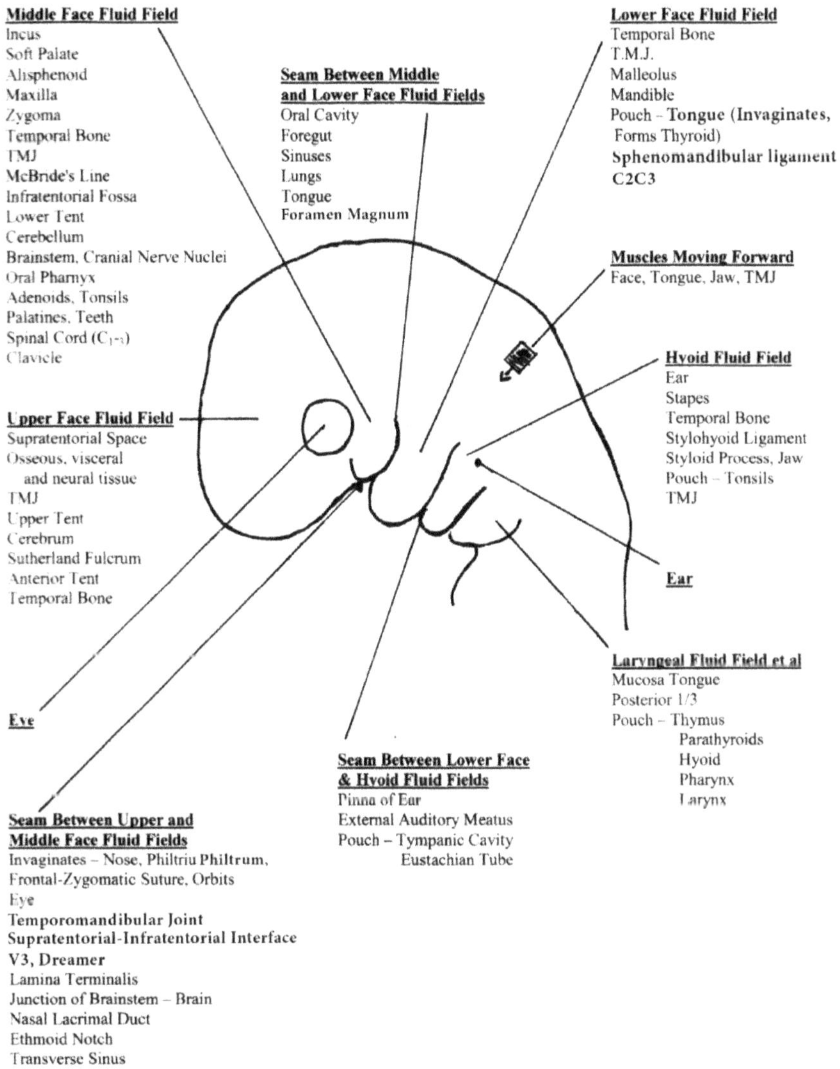


***STRUCTURES PRESENTED HERE ARE NONANATOMICAL. THEY REFER TO THE FLUID FIELDS OF GROWTH AND DEVELOPMENT FOR THAT PARTICULAR FUNCTION.***

# THE SINUSES ARE ONE SINGLE SINUS

***There is always another change we must accept in life.***
***The sinuses are a classic case of mistaken identity.***

The sinuses are named for the bones they have relationship to. We are told there are maxillary sinuses, ethmoidal sinuses, frontal sinuses, sphenoidal sinuses, mastoid sinuses (air cells) and other endothelial visceral functions (eustachian tube, middle ear) within the cranium that secrete fluids to protect the function from stasis and subsequent disease. Keeping these visceral spaces open is vital. Cranial work has added assistance for problems related to these areas. But these are not areas.

There is only one sinus.

The sinuses and all endothelial viscera of the head are a single, hollow viscus. After the lung bud opens and has momentum, the branches of the sinus tree merge together as one sinus. The seed sprouts and a single tube comes forth. It branches. The branches have names (all those listed above). The sinus tree grows for twenty-eight years, finally reaching its full image as the sphenoidal sinus opens the last branch into the dorsum sellae (just under the third ventricle where the logarithmic spiral begins). The tree grows during all the stages of life. The function of the tree is one movement that supports all sinus and ear functions.

The sinus tree has a Zone B and a transparency to the Sea Around Us.

The seam appears first and creates the enfoldments that create the branches (the individual areas). The appearance is that the branches grow out of the trunk. Growth is into the form of the space that the

Tide opens, and that is a "direction of ease." Growth depends on the seam.

The seam around the edge of the tree has three natures. Like other seams, this seam has an anatomical, a functional, and a healthy seam. The seam we want to work with is the functional seam, where we find the Long-tide and other Tidal forces. But first, let's discuss what a sinus does, then what is in the seam.

Think about what functions sinuses perform.

Think about the contents of the seam.

# THE GENERAL HISTORY OF THE SINUSES

The respiratory tree begins early. After the lungs bud at around three weeks, then the sinus tree, as I call it, buds. It grows for twenty-eight years.

The maxillary sinus begins around the third month and then the ethmoid near the fifth month, in utero. At birth these are all the sinuses we have, but other endothelial structures are forming (middle ear, eustachian tube, mastoid air cells).

After birth there is an explosion of growth. The middle face posterior cranial fossae are growing eight times faster than the upper facial fluid fields. The cerebellum is growing rapidly compared to the rest of the brain proper. The sinuses are "laid back" for a while, but around the fifth month the sphenoid sinus begins its twenty-seven-year journey to maturity.

The frontal sinuses do not move into the upper field until year five or six, after the middle face field has made major changes. This means the teeth, sinuses, oral pharynx, ear, cerebellum, brainstem, and upper neck have changed dramatically before the work is redistributed.

All this is guided by the blueprint that is invisible, unfolding via the seams which open space for new form while the old transmutes.

Sinuses get sick. The resolution depends on the reestablishment of normal functions. The movement in the whole tree is what moves each branch; therefore, we treat the whole viscera at once.

When you sense a normal sinus (whole), several involuntary motions are evident: the response to thoracic respiration and the response to Primary Respiration.

Thoracic respiration causes a general opening in all the branches. This appears as a dilation and return.

The response to Primary Respiration is metabolic motion as described in Phase One. The appearance of this is a single motion of the hollow viscus around a central fulcrum; all the branches are on the fulcrum. This is rare before treatment but is the determinant of the end point in the practical. It is amazing to see the asynchrony transmute and new elemental motion reappear, knowing what this means to the health of the sinus.

# THE PRACTICAL FOR THE SINUSES

First check the state of the whole of Zone B, and rebalance if necessary.

Sense the viscera, not the bones. Get your mind around the edges of the sinus (more or less; do not force the image, take what comes easily).

Is the viscus moving as one hollow sinus around a central fulcrum (stillness)?

Or

Is there a response to thoracic respiration?

When doing evaluations, if you do not see something easily, then it's not there. Do not push for information—it locks up the fluid body and the brainstem gets irritable (sympathetic overload). This makes the lesion field opaque, so one tries harder, and so on.

If you decide to treat, go into the seam. It will feel like space, not the space between structures, but a darkness that is empty (or so it seems).

The space may feel compressed, withered. Note this, but look for the health, for a therapeutic force already there. Soon you will find a small drop of Long-Tide waiting for you.

Synchronize with its internal tempo and intelligence.

Remember, it is a tributary of the great Sea Around Us. Open to the fulcrum for the Long-Tide. What is generating it?

After the end point, rebalance Zone B and the sea around us. Wait until you feel them connect.

# SELECTED SUMMARIES

***No. 1***

There are two Zone Bs, one that can lesion and one in the health.

There are three levels of stillness.

There are three foundational breaths: thoracic, primary and embryonic.

There is only one drop. It is in the sea.

Wholeness is the smallest division of health.

There is no distance in the mind that moves the fluid body. It is one place.

***No. 2***

*The Ontogenetic Basis of Human Differentiation*, E. Blechschmidt

*The Beginnings of Human Life*, E. Blechschmidt

*Langman's Medical Embryology*, T. Sadler

*Synchronicity*, C. Jung

*Patterns of Renewal*, L. van der Post

*The Secret of the Golden Flower*, T. Cleary

"Fulcrums," T. Schooley

*Philosophy of Osteopathy* (chapter 1), A. T. Still

***No. 3***

First breath, last breath, one breath.

Space, emptiness, crucible of creation, holy darkness.

Self dies and is taken by self into hallowed ground.

***No. 4***

The Schematic of the Osteopathic Lesion:

1. The drop from the sea, the fulcrum of form and function,

point of orientation, wholeness

2. The segmental midline
3. Motion without resistance, direction of ease
4. Physiological barrier, autonomic nervous system remains undisturbed, natural boundary of homeostasis
5. Unphysiological barrier, autonomic nervous system is disturbed, fluids begin to wither, stasis begins, symptoms are functional, early stages of disease appear, the tissues are boggy, muscles tire easily, sense of well-being declines, consciousness is aroused, therapeutic forces emerge
6. Anatomical barrier, distortion of form and function, disease begins its natural history, the functional range of motion ruptures and crescendos, metabolic inaccuracies
7. The stars and one's sense of cause, the sense of one's health, unalterable, eternal

### *No. 5*

Do not split the body in half. The right hand feels the whole and the left hand feels the whole. If the right feels the right side and the left feels the left side, then you create a false midline.

### *No. 6*

In Phase Three we learned about the dural sacs around the brain and cerebellum. These sacs juxtapose one another and create a space between the two layers of the tent. From our studies in Phase Five we can now begin to see that the space between the tents is a seam that runs all the way to the ethmoidal notch. Our sense of the space must grow as we do.

### *No. 7*

Fluid fields form and maintain bones. When the fluid field lesions, the bone deforms and continues to grow, deformed. When the fluid field is able to go to neutral, the original form begins to express itself.

### *No. 8*

The cranial vertebral junction is at C3. This is where the epidural space begins. The atlas and axis both are intracranial during the early days of growth. The C1/C2 nerves innervate the cerebellar sac (lower tent). The idea that the neck begins at C3 was a common theme in the time when I was studying with Dr. Wales.

### *No. 9*

We begin treatment with stillness and we end with stillness.

### *No. 10*

Blows to the occiput lock up fluid fields in the middle face. The fulcrum holding the lesion could be in the front.

We evolve in our skill not through removing lesions,
but by what we learn at end points.

# BIODYNAMICS OF OSTEOPATHY BOOK SERIES

This book is one of a series of twelve *Biodynamics of Osteopathy* books. It is recommended that you read the whole series in order, as each book builds on the understanding from prior books. It is also recommended that you seek experienced teachers and mentors to help you experience the full depth of the information given.

The full series is as follows:

**Phase One** is about involuntary motion, which is motion present in the whole and in the lesion. We learn to synchronize with the breathing of Primary Respiration before we approach any treatment. This synchronization is the key to working with stable rates and not irritating the system. The principle of synchronizing with a healthy aspect of the patient suffuses the whole teaching program. This synchronization shifts our awareness to a different level of receptivity, which allows us to see Primary Respiration rather than the lesion field, and this eventually leads us to an understanding of the intention of Primary Respiration.

**Phase Two** is about communication with the natural laws of healing that surround activity at 2 to 3 cycles per minute. We synchronize with the breathing of Primary Respiration and also add the skill of sensing the fulcrum, the Stillness through which the breathing creates form and function. It is a different kind of synchronization from that in Phase One, shifting our awareness more deeply. As this occurs, the treatment automatically expresses itself. The end point of treatment, when compared with Phase One, reveals several differences. We find this kind of synchronization works exclusively with the fluid body and the outcome of treatment is more complete than when working with tissue alone.

**Phase Three** is centered around the activities of the Long Tide (100 second cycle). We explore an indwelling therapeutic force already present in the lesion field. We learn that the dural system is not made-up of three sickles but rather a series of folds in a sac, arising during growth and development. We see the relationship between the upper and lower dural sacs, awakening us to the independence of two separate tentorium cerebelli. We discover that zone D, the horizon, and the Wire (along which the Long Tide moves during its intended therapeutic course) are all linked as natural laws pertaining to this level of Primary Respiration.

**Phase Four** focuses on the Midline, a place where the spatial relationships are expressed as a whole. It synchronizes and centers us in such a way that we become aware of Zone D and the Dynamic Stillness. The Third Level Stillness in Phase Four is different from the Stillness in the other Phases – we are centered by the Stillness at the center of creation. Our intention is replaced by the intention of the Tide which can facilitate our spiritual path.

**Phase Five** is about *the face.* As we approach the face, we use all of the principles that we have learned in Phase One, Two, Three, and Four. We work with automatic shifting and notice differences from how the face is viewed by older models within Osteopathy in the Cranial Field. As we synchronize with the therapeutic presence of the Long Tide we see what we can learn about the face from that landscape. We also work with Seams, Dynamic Stillness, and Ignition.

**Phase Six** is a continuation of our journey into the Wholeness that generates life and delivers therapeutic forces that transmute lesions once Neutral is expressed. It is a mixture of activities centered around the outside presence of Primary Respiration as something that is a non-biological force and that has a persona. We will also continue to explore seams and then move on to the extremities, first in the embryological terms and then as Sutherland taught them in his work called PowerPoints. Phase 6 is a time to build your understanding of the Tide and refine your skills.

**Phase Seven** highlights the Health. Dr. Still's famous comment "Find the Health; anyone can find disease," has plagued many minds over the last century. We come to the clear vision of several indwelling aspects of the Health: Love ... liquid light ... and a diamond matrix. A approach to the terminally ill and dying patient is addressed. In the somatic sensation of the Tide passing through the House Under the Sea, our awareness is transmuted by the Health. The lesion is seen as a precognitive act of the Health. Thoracic Respiration, Primary Respiration, and Ignition are as One. The landscape is vast ... and the principles of healing are even more substantial than we have previously experienced..

**Phase Eight** is a deeper exploration of seams, balanced rhythmic interchange, and the Flame of Intention as a therapeutic modality. Phase Eight is the culmination of our awareness of Wholeness, and ultimately brings us to the Divine Presence, Unconditional Love and Oneness. The living Tide dominates the awareness while forms move to the background. One feels the Breath of Creation in oneself as the Center of Wholeness. One feels the Unfoldment of oneself as one is Created. Our consciousness is a gift; we do not own it and if we try to control it we lose Wholeness.

**Phase Nine** is when we are able to fully evaluate and treat the

Central Nervous System and the Eye. We also address Fire and the therapeutic modality of the Shakedown. True action is moved from Love and makes our perception exist. This Love is self-emptying and by its nature allows us to Serve as part of the Perfect. Perception can be used to Serve something other than ourselves. We have attempted to enter this balance point between the Perfect and the Disease ... it is a point where the whole of everything is suspended by Love as it works to incarnate the Complete. In the balance point of everything is The Intention of the Tide following the movement of the distortion back to a True relationship with the Blueprint of Life.

**Pediatrics One** explores how children grow as a whole, not in parts as we sometimes believe. Children live in the Direction of Ease of motion present in their fluid metabolic fields, otherwise they get uncomfortable and require assistance. Does your treatment directly support the whole, or does it assume to support the whole? We realize children are not adults and cannot be treated as adults are. We approach the therapeutic modality of the "Meeting Place", prenatal and postnatal periods, the treatment of the pelvis during pregnancy, fetal malposition and labor.

**Pediatrics Two** is where we deepen in the perceptive awareness necessary to approach the treatment of children. We deepen in our appreciation of Wholeness, the three levels of Stillness and the "Meeting Place". We approach "Desert Neutral", where therapeutics pass into the neutral substance, and a mystery unfolds as the breath of Divine love cascades as a therapeutic force across a night desert landscape, filling and leaving behind no visible effects. We further address treatment of the pelvis and the uterus during pregnancy. We explore thoracic and Primary Respiration in children, and the Family Circle.

**Pediatrics Three** is where we continue to study the therapeutic

Flow of Attention. We deepen in Third Level Stillness and the Meeting Place. The Meeting Place is easily misinterpreted ... our observer must be so still and neutral that the process can be seen as it happens. The central nervous system in the child can be finally approached for evaluation and treatment. We explore teething and also the "locked up head". We use the therapeutic modality of the Flame of Intention, and its connection to the Breath of Life. Everything is transparent to the Breath of Life.

# ABOUT THE AUTHOR

James Jealous, D.O. (1943–2021), was an osteopathic physician, teacher, and writer. His life's work was founding and developing **Biodynamics of Osteopathy**, a unique methodology he established within the field of osteopathy, following the lineage of Dr. A.T. Still and Dr. W.G. Sutherland.

He was born in Saco, Maine, and since his father was an osteopathic physician, he was around osteopathy from an early age. He studied at Kirksville College of Osteopathic Medicine in Missouri (now the A.T. Still University of Health Sciences), graduating in 1970. He then set up practice in rural Maine as an osteopathic primary care physician.

Over time, Dr. Jealous saw parallels between the work of embryologist Dr. Erich Blechschmidt and that of osteopathic physician Dr. William Garner Sutherland. This inspiration led him to create his own body of work. In the early 1990s, he began teaching "A Biodynamic View of Osteopathy in the Cranial Field," which, as he developed his specific methodology, was refined to "Biodynamics of Osteopathy."

A deeply spiritual person, he felt most at home in the natural world and was an avid fisherman and hiker.

For more information, please visit:
**https://BiodynamicsOfOsteopathy.com**

There is a wind passing through ...
it is the motion of creation,
the eternal motion of Divine love.

www.ingramcontent.com/pod-product-compliance
Lightning Source LLC
LaVergne TN
LVHW071339210926
848486LV00003B/189
* 9 7 9 8 2 9 5 5 3 9 2 8 2 *